# DIABETI

# JUICING

## FOR

# SENIORS

**21 Tasty Renal - Friendly Juice Recipe to Regulate Blood Sugar, Balance Electrolyte, Detoxify, Improve Kidney Function and Prevent Dialysis**

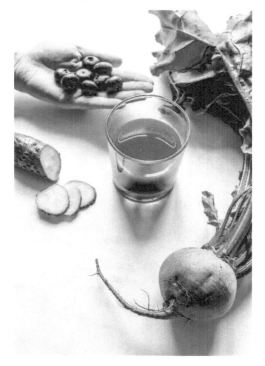

## DR. AGISA BEGAY

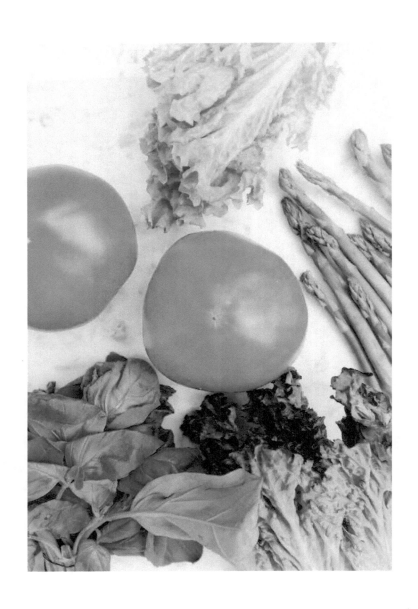

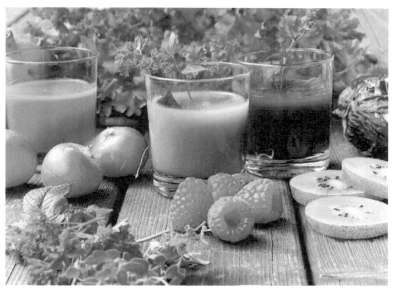

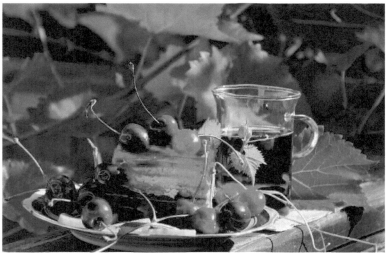

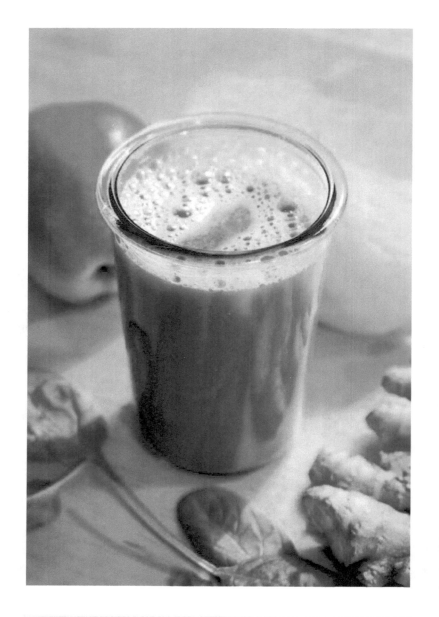

# Dedication

*This book **"Diabetic Renal Juicing for Seniors"** is dedicated to each and every senior out there fighting for survival. May this book bring forth a renewed hope in yourhealing journey.*

*This book is a work of **"personalized experience"** and it will surely be a guide to your wellness.*

# Table of Contents

Introduction ...................................................... 13

A Survivor's Story ......................................... 13

Symptoms.................................................. 21

Causes of Diabetic Renal Disease ................................ 22

Chapter One ...................................................... 25

Diabetes' Role in Kidney Disease ................................ 25

Tips for Maintaining Kidney Health.............................. 25

Diabetes and Kidney Failure..................................... 27

Risk Factors.................................................. 27

Complications................................................. 28

Diabetic Kidney Disease Prevention............................. 29

Chapter Two...................................................... 33

Getting Started in the Juicing World ............................ 33

Advantages of juicing on your blood sugar levels and kidney health ................................................ 33

Selecting the Best Juicer........................................ 35

What to Avoid When Juicing with Kidney Disease........ 35

What fruits and vegetables should diabetic renal disease patients consume? ........................................ 37

Juices with Low Potassium ............................... 38

Recipe 1 .................................................. 39

Ingredients ................................................................ 39

Preparation ............................................................... 40

Recipe 2 ................................................................... 41

Ingredients ................................................................ 41

Preparations .............................................................. 42

Recipe 3 ................................................................... 42

Ingredients ................................................................ 43

Preparation ............................................................... 44

Recipe 4 ................................................................... 45

Ingredients ................................................................ 45

Preparation ............................................................... 45

Recipe 5 ................................................................... 48

Ingredients ................................................................ 48

Preparation ............................................................... 49

Recipe 6 ................................................................... 51

Ingredients ................................................................ 52

Preparations .............................................................. 52

Recipe 7 ................................................................... 55

Ingredients ................................................................ 55

Preparations .............................................................. 55

Recipe 8 ................................................................... 57

Preparations .............................................................. 58

Recipe 9 ...................................................................... 59

Ingredients ................................................................. 60

Preparation ................................................................ 60

Recipe 10 ................................................................... 61

Ingredients ................................................................. 62

Preparation ................................................................ 62

Recipe 11 ................................................................... 64

Ingredients ................................................................. 64

Preparation ................................................................ 65

Recipe 12 ................................................................... 66

Ingredients ................................................................. 67

Preparation ................................................................ 67

Recipe 13 ................................................................... 69

Ingredients ................................................................. 69

Preparations ............................................................... 70

Recipe 14 ................................................................... 72

Ingredients ................................................................. 72

Preparation ................................................................ 73

Recipe 15 ................................................................... 74

Ingredients ................................................................. 74

Preparation ................................................................ 75

Recipe 16 ................................................................... 75

Ingredients ................................................................ 76

Preparation ............................................................. 76

Recipe 17 ................................................................ 77

Ingredients ............................................................. 77

Preparation ............................................................. 77

Recipe 18 ................................................................ 79

Ingredients ............................................................. 79

Preparation ............................................................. 80

Recipe 19 ................................................................ 81

Ingredients ............................................................. 82

Preparation ............................................................. 82

Recipe 20 ................................................................ 84

Ingredients ............................................................. 84

Preparation ............................................................. 85

Recipe 21 ................................................................ 86

Ingredients ............................................................. 87

Preparation ............................................................. 87

Bonus 1 ................................................................... 89

21-Day Diabetic Kidney Disease Meal Plan ................... 89

WEEK 1 ................................................................ 89

WEEK 2 ................................................................ 92

WEEK 3 ................................................................ 95

Conclusion ........................................................ 98

Bonus 2 .......................................................... 100

   Food Journal .............................................. 100

Picture Links ................................................... 120

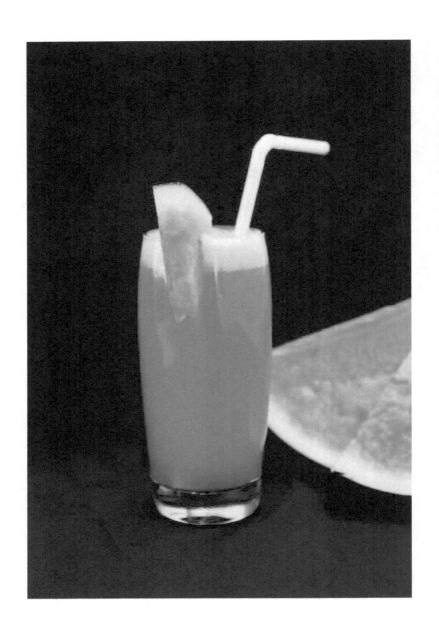

# Introduction

## A Survivor's Story

Jane Robinson spent most afternoons as a child growing up in Texas with a group of her neighborhood pals. They preferred conversing around the picnic table to playing on the playground or watching sports, and they would sip sodas and eat junk food as they talked.

"We were never really taught about fitness or nutrition and, unfortunately, those same habits transferred into adult life," Jane says. "When I first started working, if I was hungry, I'd get fast food, chips, or a soda." And I continued failing to exercise."

Jane had no idea her decisions were endangering her health, especially considering both her mother and grandmother were diabetes. Many years later, she recognizes the value of proper nutrition and exercise. She also acknowledges the need of self-care for physical and mental well-being and wishes for others to benefit from her experience.

"You've got to make time for yourself," she insists. "That is essential for self-love. You need to calm down and prioritize your needs."

Jane was diagnosed with diabetes in 2005, despite her poor diet and family history. However, as a single mother with a school-aged child, she couldn't afford the time and money spent on prescriptions and doctor appointments.

"I wasn't feeling sick, and it was more important to go to work and take care of the bills," Jane says. "It was either pay for healthcare or feed my child."

Jane suffered from chronic migraine headaches (a diabetes symptom) for several years but had no idea why. She took excessive amounts of over-the-counter pain relievers without realizing they were damaging to her kidneys. Jane didn't feel knowledgeable enough to ask concerns regarding her kidney health until she could afford to see a doctor. She did almost little to better her condition since she didn't know what else to do—a mistake she later regretted.

Jane discovered her kidney function was extremely low in 2013. She was meant to see a nephrologist, but she was in the process of relocating, so the move and job search took precedence.

Jane's health continued to deteriorate after she relocated to Houston. Her best friend drove her to an area hospital's emergency room one trying night. There, she found a caring doctor who agreed to accept Jane as a patient despite the fact that she had no insurance at the moment. He told Jane about end-stage renal illness, how dialysis would make her feel better if her health condition worsened, and persuaded her to try dieting and juicing.

Concerns about her work schedule and not having enough time to prepare these dishes made her hesitant to begin these juice treatments. But she soon found herself with little choice. Jane told a friend about the doctor's advise to buy a juicing book written by the well-known Dr. Agisa Begay, as this book will help her make these healthy juices with ease.

Jane quickly obtained a copy of this book and began using the recipes in it; she didn't have any strange feelings about the taste of the recipes because they all tasted really good, which was contrary to what she had thought all along; she had assumed that these juices would be tasteless, but to her greatest surprise, her taste buds were loving these delights as the day progressed. "It's been three months since I started my juicing therapy, and it's really changed her life," Jane said, adding that she's taking more vacations, socializing more, and no longer requires her daughter (now 19) to come over and help with cleaning. Jane has also progressed from requesting favors from her mother to granting them.

"My mom saw the difference in my energy, and started asking me to drive her around, instead of the opposite," she says while grinning.

Jane is grateful to have her life back now that she is taking better care of herself. She exercises often and has worked with a dietitian to ensure she is eating healthily. She's lost a lot of weight thanks to these delectable treats. Her aims are to continue decreasing weight, stay healthy, and avoid dialysis as much as possible.

Despite her difficulties, Jane considers herself fortunate and takes every chance to give back. She assists special needs persons in participating in various activities and educates others about the benefits of juicing and the hazards of diabetes as a patient advocate.

"It's so important to educate yourself about health issues," Jane explains. "I discovered too late that diabetes can be a silent killer." I didn't have any of the symptoms. Many persons with diabetes may not feel well or do not want to confess they are ill. 'Look at me,' I say. I'll serve as an example. Take good care of oneself and never ignore diabetes."

In the complicated process of treating diabetes, most people seek natural, holistic remedies that can help them fight this terrible health condition. Fruits and vegetables are laced with potent elixirs that offer a ray of hope to diabetic renal disease sufferers.

Welcome to *"Diabetic Renal Juicing for Seniors"* a thorough handbook that reveals nature's incredible possibilities for diabetic management and renal health.

Diabetes is a serious health problem that poses a substantial danger, and diabetic renal disease is a concerning consequence produced by the disease's mismanagement. Many people have found the medicinal properties of fruits and vegetables over the course of time but they are still bewildered about the complexities of juicing. Unfortunately, juicing is commonly misunderstood, and its benefits are sometimes overshadowed. We understand your concerns, and our goal with this book is to elucidate the route to healthy juicing for those with diabetic renal illness.

Our book is your dependable companion on this wellness journey. We will demystify the art of juicing in the following chapters, taking you through the complexities of selecting, preparing, and extracting the most effective juices to promote your wellness.

We pledge to fill the information gap by providing you with a thorough grasp of how fruits and vegetables can be used to help control diabetes. Our book will introduce you to a variety of flavors that can benefit your health, from the vivid sweetness of berries to the earthy deliciousness of leafy greens.

**"Diabetic Renal Juicing for Seniors"** is more than simply a book; it's a life-changing event. It's a trip that will provide you with the knowledge to make informed decisions, transforming natural elements into powerful tools in your fight against diabetic renal disease. Join us on this revitalizing adventure as we explore the extraordinary power of nature's juices to improve your well-being and provide hope to your diabetes control path.

Before we delve into juicing, it will be proper we raise our awareness about this disease.

Diabetic renal disease also known as Diabetic nephropathy is a severe consequence of both type 1 and type 2 diabetes. It occurs when prolonged high blood sugar levels associated with diabetes damage the small blood vessels in the kidneys. Over time, this damage can lead to kidney dysfunction and, in severe cases, kidney failure. It is one of the leading causes of end-stage renal disease (ESRD) or kidney failure in people with diabetes. One in every three diabetics in the United States suffers from diabetic nephropathy.

Diabetic nephropathy impairs the kidneys' capacity to perform their normal function of eliminating waste products and excess fluid from the body. Maintaining a healthy lifestyle and properly treating your diabetes and high blood pressure are the greatest ways to prevent or delay diabetic nephropathy.

Over time, the condition wreaks havoc on your kidneys' sensitive filtering function. Early treatment may prevent or decrease the progression of the disease and lessen the likelihood of consequences.

Renal disease can lead to renal failure, commonly known as end-stage kidney disease. Kidney failure is a potentially fatal disorder. Dialysis or a kidney transplant are the only therapy options at this point.

**Symptoms**

You would most likely not notice any signs or symptoms of diabetic nephropathy in the early stages. Signs and symptoms in the later stages may include:

- Improving blood pressure regulation

- Protein in urine

- Foot, ankle, hand, or eye swelling

- Increased desire to urinate

- Less reliance on insulin or diabetes medication

- Disorientation or difficulty concentrating

- Breathing difficulties


- Appetite loss

- Vomiting and nausea

- Constant itching

- Tiredness


## Causes of Diabetic Renal Disease

Diabetic renal disease is a common type 1 and type 2 diabetic consequence. Diabetes damages blood vessels and other kidney cells, resulting in diabetic renal disease. This occurs due to various factors, primarily driven by long-term high blood sugar levels. The key causes include:

- **Hyperglycemia:** Having prolonged elevated blood sugar levels tend to damage the small blood vessels (capillaries) in the kidneys, impairing their function.

- **High Blood Pressure:** Hypertension have been shown to be a common comorbidity in diabetics and contributes to kidney damage by further straining blood vessels.

- **Genetics:** Hereditary factor can come to play as some individuals may be genetically predisposed to diabetic renal disease, making them more susceptible to kidney damage.

- **Smoking and Obesity:** Lifestyle factors such as smoking and obesity can exacerbate the risk.

# Chapter One

## Diabetes' Role in Kidney Disease

Each kidney is made up of millions of small filters called nephrons. Elevated blood sugar can damage blood arteries in the kidneys as well as nephrons over time, causing them to function less effectively. Many diabetics develop excessive blood pressure, which can also harm the kidneys.

CKD takes a long time to develop and typically has no symptoms in the early stages. Unless your doctor tests you, you won't know if you have CKD.

## Tips for Maintaining Kidney Health

Controlling your blood sugar, blood pressure, and cholesterol levels can help keep your kidneys healthy. High levels of blood sugar, blood pressure, and cholesterol are all risk factors for heart disease and stroke. Following the tips below will not only keep you in check for diabetics, it will as well prevented other disease that possess high chances of manifesting as a result of diabetics, endeavor you;

• Try to keep your blood sugar levels as close to normal as possible.

• Get an A1C test at least twice a year, and more frequently if your medication changes or if you have other health issues. Consult your doctor about how frequently you should exercise.

• Check your blood pressure on a daily basis and keep it below 140/90 mm/Hg (or the target given by your doctor). Consult your doctor about blood pressure medications and other options.

• Maintain your desired cholesterol level.

• Consume low-sodium foods.

• Consume more fruits and vegetables.

• Engage in physical activity.

• Take your medications exactly as prescribed.

## Diabetes and Kidney Failure

Taking measures to prevent type 2 diabetes if you have prediabetes is a critical step in preventing kidney disease. According to research, people who are overweight and at a higher risk of getting type 2 diabetes can prevent or delay the disease by decreasing 5% to 7% of their body weight, or 10 to 14 pounds for a person weighing 200 pounds. You can accomplish this by eating healthier and engaging in 150 minutes of physical activity every week. The National Diabetes Prevention Program lifestyle change program of the CDC can assist you in developing the healthy lifestyle behaviors required to prevent type 2 diabetes. Programs as such are very valuable, especially for a diabetic patient.

## Risk Factors

Factors that can raise your risk of diabetic nephropathy if you have diabetes include:

• Hyperglycemia (uncontrolled high blood sugar)

• Hypertension (uncontrolled high blood pressure)

• Having a smoking habit

• Hypercholesterolemia

• Obesity.

• A family history of Diabetes and renal disease.

## Complications

Complications of diabetic renal disease may develop gradually over months or years. They may include:

• Fluid retention, which can cause arm and leg swelling, high blood pressure, or fluid in the lungs (pulmonary edema).

• An elevated blood potassium levels (hyperkalemia)

• Cardiovascular illness (heart and blood vessel disease), which can lead to stroke

• Diabetes retinopathy (damage to the blood vessels of the light-sensitive tissue at the rear of the eye)

• A decrease in the amount of red blood cells that transport oxygen (anemia)

• Foot ulcers, erectile dysfunction, diarrhea, and other symptoms of nerve and blood vessel damage

• Bone and mineral diseases caused by the kidneys' inability to maintain the proper calcium and phosphorus balance in the blood

• Pregnancy problems pose risks to both the mother and the developing fetus.

• Irreversible kidney deterioration (end-stage renal disease), requiring dialysis or a kidney transplant for survival.

## Diabetic Kidney Disease Prevention

The following guidelines should be followed correctly to lower your chance of getting diabetic nephropathy:

• Attend diabetes management appointments on a regular basis. Maintain annual appointments — or more frequent appointments if your health care provider recommends it — to assess your diabetes management and to test for diabetic nephropathy and other complications.

• Manage your diabetes. Diabetic nephropathy can be avoided or delayed with proper diabetes management.

• Manage hypertension or other medical disorders. If you have high blood pressure or other factors that put you at risk for kidney disease, work with your doctor to get them under control.

• Stick to the directions on over-the-counter drugs. Nonprescription pain remedies such as aspirin and nonsteroidal anti-inflammatory drugs such as naproxen (Aleve) and ibuprofen (Advil, Motrin IB, and others) should be taken according to the directions. Taking these types of pain medicines can cause kidney damage in patients with diabetic nephropathy.

• Keep a healthy weight. If you're already at a healthy weight, try to keep it there by being physically active most days of the week. If you need to reduce weight, talk to your doctor about weight-loss measures include increasing your daily physical activity and eating less calories.

• Quit smoking. Cigarette smoking can harm your kidneys and aggravate pre-existing renal problems. If you're a smoker, talk to your doctor about quitting methods. Support groups, counseling, and some drugs can all help you quit smoking.

If you have read to this stage of our book, it translates that you really care about your kidney. In the next chapter of this book, we will delve into the world of fruit and vegetable juicing, these juices are proven to manage your elevated blood levels, retard the progression of kidney disease, thus, helping you avoid dialysis.

*I hope you are enjoying your read so far? We are happy to be part of your wellness journey, we kindly ask you to drop a polite review in the website about how you feel using this book, as this will help us tailor our subsequent publications to meet your needs, thank you.*

# Chapter Two

## Getting Started in the Juicing World

Juicing is more popular than ever among health-conscious people, and for good reason. Juicing is the best way to get more nutrients with less work and a delicious taste. People with chronic kidney illness, on the other hand, should carefully evaluate their juicing options and ensure they are doing it right while keeping watch on their potassium, and phosphorus intake.

## Advantages of juicing on your blood sugar levels and kidney health

Juicing with diabetic kidney disease should be part of a bigger fruit and vegetable landscape, but it still has numerous health and flavor benefits that are worth investigating. Drinking fresh juice provides you with:

• Increased vitamin, mineral, and phytonutrient concentrations

• An excellent method to incorporate fruits and vegetables into your diet if you dislike them.

• The ability to develop your own flavor combinations (which can also enable you sneak in vegetables you don't like with those you enjoy)

• A higher antioxidant concentration, which can minimize inflammation, which can aggravate CKD.

• Higher nutritional contents than pasteurized juices or juices that have been stored for an extended period of time.

• Getting more plant-based foods into your diet is vital for someone with CKD, and juicing is a great method to do so, especially if you have hunger concerns as a result of the kidney disease.

## Selecting the Best Juicer

Anything that increases the amount of plants in your diet can benefit someone with diabetes and renal problems. However, blending may provide a tiny advantage over juicing. A cold press juicer provides a higher concentration of several nutrients but excludes fiber. While juicing provides more antioxidants per ounce, it also provides more of the substances you want to avoid, such as potassium.

Another item to think about is hydration intake. Because people with CKD must be cautious about the amount of fluid they consume, condensing your fruit and vegetable diet into liquid form may not be as healthful as producing a smoothie in the blender. Finally, blending provides all of the benefits of fruit consumption while also preserving additional nutrients that your body requires.

## What to Avoid When Juicing with Kidney Disease

Juicing has a lot to offer. However, like with any dietary decision with diabetic renal illness, you must use caution. Juicing has a few disadvantages, including:

- Fiber content loss

- Increased sugar consumption per ounce

- Fluid administration

- Higher levels of chemicals that can affect the kidneys

The good news is that with the right juicing knowledge and juice selection techniques you can enjoy a more healthy and smarter juicing.

Keep in Mind:

- Exercise caution while eating dark green vegetables such as spinach or kale. They include a lot of vitamin K, which can help with blood clotting. If you are on dialysis, you may not want increased clotting.

- Avoid canned vegetables, which may be heavy in salt. Alternatively, check for canned vegetables with no added sodium, or rinse them before using.

- Avoid juicing potassium-rich fruits and vegetables; this will be even more concentrated in juice form.

However, juicing has proven to be one of the best strategies to prevent diabetic kidney disease from progressing to a condition of utter health disaster, if done correctly.

As you continue reading, we will delve into kidney friendly juicing recipes and meal preps that will be beneficial in controlling diabetic kidney disorders.

### What fruits and vegetables should diabetic renal disease patients consume?

Diabetic Renal disease patients should look for low-potassium elements in fruits and vegetables such as apples, cranberries, blackberries, peaches, and pineapple. Additionally, pay attention to juice safety by thoroughly washing produce before juicing.

Try adding herbs like mint or ginger, as well as spices like cinnamon or nutmeg, for extra flavor and nutrients. It's crucial to remember that many store-bought fruit drinks are rich in sugar and should be avoided if you have kidney disease.

Note: When making any dietary changes, it's recommended to see your doctor first, followed by working with a certified dietitian who can give specialized meal plans tailored to your specific needs.

## Juices with Low Potassium

Individuals with diabetic renal disease should be cautious of their potassium consumption, since excess potassium can be hazardous to their health.

When the kidneys are not working properly, they may be unable to eliminate extra potassium from the body, resulting in hyperkalemia. Hyperkalemia can

Low potassium drinks can be a great alternative for those with kidney disease since they give hydration and important minerals without raising blood potassium levels.

Apple, cranberry, and grape juices are examples of low potassium juices. These juices can help balance electrolytes and avoid dehydration during physical activity (exercise for a healthy heart) or hot weather.

Low potassium juices, with so many delicious varieties available, provide lots of methods to keep your kidneys healthy while still enjoying your favorite drinks!

## *Recipe 1*:

### Cucumber Juice

Cucumbers have a high water content but a low potassium concentration. Cucumber juice is also high in vitamin K and antioxidants.

## *Ingredients*

- 1 large English cucumber (about 1 to 1/2 standard cucumbers)
- 1 apple, green
- 1 cup of water
- 12 tsp lemon or lime juice (optional)

## Preparation

• Peel the cucumber if using a regular cucumber (no need to peel an English cucumber!). Chop the cucumber roughly. Chop the apple while leaving the skin on.

• In a blender, combine the cucumber, apple, and water. Blend on high until the mixture is pureed and a liquid forms.

• Strain the juice through a fine mesh sieve or a nut milk bag to remove any pulp. Discard the pulp (or use as suggested above). Add the fresh lemon or lime juice (more if required). Drink immediately over ice, or cool first.

**Notes:**

- Use English cucumber since the juice may be made without peeling the cucumber.

- Cabbage juice contains a high concentration of vitamins K, C, B6, and B9. Cabbage is also a high-fiber food.

## Recipe 2

**Celery Juice:**

Celery is high in antioxidants, has anti-inflammatory properties, and aids digestion.

All of these juices contain important vitamins and minerals that can benefit your general health and well-being.

## Ingredients

- 8 medium-sized celery stalks (approximately 1 bunch)
- 1 medium green apple

- 12 cup of water

- Optional: 1 teaspoon lemon or lime juice

## Preparations

• Finely cut the celery. Chop the apple while leaving the skin on.

• In a blender, combine the celery, apple, and water. Blend on high until the mixture is pureed and a liquid forms.

• Strain the juice through a fine mesh sieve or a nut milk bag to remove any pulp. Discard the pulp (or use as suggested above). Add the fresh lemon juice (more if desired). Drink immediately over ice, or cool first.

## Recipe 3:

### Cranberries Juice

Cranberry contains a high concentration of vitamin C, vitamin E, vitamin B2, vitamin B3, vitamin B1, vitamin B9, vitamin B6, vitamin K, and vitamin A. If you have diabetic kidney disease, you should know that drinking cranberry juice may help prevent UTIs due to its antimicrobial qualities.

People who drink cranberry juice had lower levels of low-density lipoprotein (LDL), also known as "bad" cholesterol. This suggests that cranberry juice may be advantageous to your heart health as well.

## *Ingredients*

• 2 cups fresh or frozen cranberries

• 2 cups distilled water

• 1 1/2 tbsp lemon juice or orange juice (optional); lemon juice for low vitamin A levels

• 1 sprinkle raw honey or maple syrup, stevia, or your preferred sweetener (optional)

## Preparation

• In a blender, combine cranberries and water and blend on high for 2 minutes.

• Check to see if there are any solid cranberry bits left, and if so, blend until they are gone.

• Pass through a fine mesh screen or cheesecloth to strain.

• If preferred, add lemon or orange juice and sweetener. I like mine unsweetened, although it may be too sour for certain people.

• The juice can be stored in the refrigerator for a few days.

- If you have a high-speed blender and don't mind pulp in your juice, skip the straining step and enjoy the full cranberry flavor!

*Recipe 4*

**Grape Juice**

*Ingredients*

- 4–8 pounds fresh harvested grapes (Concord grapes)

*Preparation*

- Gather a large basket, put on long sleeves and a cap, bring clippers, and fill it with grape bunches.

- Remember that 1 pound of grapes yields slightly less than 1 cup of juice.

- Place the grapes in a basin of water. Then rinse the individual grapes, pulling them away from the stem, placing them in a wide bowl, and discarding the green, unripe, and old shriveled grapes.

- Mash the grapes with a potato masher until the juice starts to flow. If you have a large number of grapes to harvest, you may need to work in batches. We've discovered that mash roughly 4 pounds of grapes at a time works best.

- Transfer the crushed grapes to a large stockpot. Bring the grapes and juice to a boil over medium heat and cook for 10 minutes.. Stir frequently to prevent the grapes from sticking to the bottom of the pan. Mash some more halfway through cooking, breaking up as many of the leftover grapes as possible.

- Get another large pot and cover it with a fine mesh screen. Alternatively, wrap it in two layers of cheesecloth and bind it with a rubber band. Place the saucepan on a plate to catch any juice that may spill.

- Strain the grape mixture through a fine mesh strainer or cheesecloth. Allow to strain for several hours or overnight in the refrigerator.

- Take out the sieve or cheesecloth. Take note that sediment will have accumulated on the container's bottom. Rinse the sieve or cheesecloth and sift the juice again to remove any remaining debris. Fill containers with juice by pouring or ladling it. Have fun with your juice!

Helpful Tip:

It should be noted that the grape mash can be composted.

After about a week in the fridge, I notice that the juice begins to ferment, which isn't necessarily a negative thing; it just adds some natural carbonation. If you leave it for too long, it will eventually turn to vinegar. This is why we strive to make only as much as we'll need in one week.

## Recipe 5

### Blueberry Juice

Berries are an excellent choice for juice, and blueberries are especially beneficial to individuals with renal diabetes due to their lower potassium level than other fruits. Here's a simple homemade blueberry juice recipe that's helpful for persons with kidney diabetes; it's one of my favorites, and I'd love for you to try it:

## Ingredients:

• 2 cups of blueberries, fresh or frozen (thawed if frozen)

• 1/2 to 1 cup water (adjust according to taste)

• 1-2 tablespoons lemon juice (optional, for added flavor)

• 1-2 teaspoons sugar substitute (optional; choose a diabetic-friendly sugar alternative)

*Preparation*:

- If you're using fresh blueberries, rinse them thoroughly in cold water and remove any stems or leaves.

- If using frozen blueberries, thaw them according to package recommendations.

- Combine the blueberries in a blender or food processor.

- Begin by adding 1/2 cup of water. You can then add extra water to achieve the required juice consistency.

- For a somewhat tangy flavor, add 1-2 teaspoons lemon juice to the blender.

- Blend the ingredients until they form a smooth purée. If the mixture is too thick, add more water gradually and blend until the desired consistency is achieved.

- Strain the juice by placing a fine mesh sieve or cheesecloth over a large basin or pitcher.

- Strain the blueberry puree through a sieve to separate the juice from the pulp and seeds. To extract as much juice as possible, knead the mixture with a spoon or spatula.

- Serve the blueberry juice immediately in a glass or container, with or without ice.

- Any leftover juice can be refrigerated and used later. Store in an airtight jar and use within a few days.

For diabetic renal sufferers, this low-potassium homemade blueberry juice could be a delicious and kidney-friendly treatment. Adjust the sweetness and consistency to your liking to effectively balance blood sugar levels, and be mindful of portion proportions. Always get expert nutritional guidance from a healthcare provider or dietitian based on your unique health requirements.

## *Recipe 6*

**Pineapple Juice Recipe**

Pineapple juice, the most nutrient-dense fruit juice, offers numerous health benefits due to its high concentration of minerals, fibre, enzymes, vitamin C, and energy. The method utilized in this juicing recipe helps to keep all of the nutritional fibers and nutrients that would otherwise be lost in its canned equivalent. Aside from the health advantages, this dish includes black pepper and very little salt, which lend a lovely salty-spicy zing to the sweet taste.

## Ingredients:

- 1/2 cup chopped Fresh Pineapple
- Optional: a sprinkle of ground black pepper
- 1-2 teaspoon sugar (optional)
- Optional pinch of salt
- 1 cup of water
- 5-6 cubes of ice

## Preparations:

- Wash the pineapple and use a large knife to remove the outer skin. It should be cut in half. Chop one half into small pieces. Keep the other half for another use. If you don't want to peel it, you can use shop purchased pineapple (we recommend sliced fresh pineapple). If you're using pineapple slices, cut them and measure out 1/2 cup chopped pieces.

- Fill a blender or mixer grinder jar halfway with water. Mix in the pineapple chunks.

- Blend until the puree is smooth and there are no bits of fruit.

- Place a fine mesh sieve over a large bowl and pour in the prepared puree.

- Gently press it with a spatula to extract as much juice as possible from the pulp. Remove any remaining pulp.

- Stir in the ice cubes for a minute. Taste the juice and season with sugar, salt, and black pepper powder to taste. After a minute of stirring, pour it into two serving glasses and serve.

## Tips and Variations:

- If you wish to produce cold pineapple juice, place the chopped pineapple in the refrigerator before using.

- The ripe pineapple is essential to the success of this recipe. Select one with golden yellow to brown skin. Avoid pineapple with green or dark brown skin. It will have a strong sweet smell if it is ripe.

- Adjust the amount of sugar or use other sugar alternatives to taste.

- You can also use a juicer to make the juice.

*Recipe 7*

**Watermelon Juice Recipe**

Watermelon juice is best consumed on hot summer days since it instantly cools the body and fills it with water and minerals lost through sweating. This ultimate thirst quencher fresh fruit juice is simple to create at home.

*Ingredients*:

- 4 cups seeded and diced watermelon (equivalent to 1 small watermelon)
- Half a lime juice
- 4 cubes of ice

*Preparations*:

- Cut the watermelon into large chunks and remove the skin. Remove the black seeds; there is no need to remove the white seeds.

- Place watermelon chunks in a blender jar.

- Blend until the texture is smooth. Mix in the lime juice in a large mixing bowl. Pour prepared watermelon juice over 1 ice cube in each serving glass.

Tips and Variations:

- To make it slushy, combine crushed ice with the remaining ingredients.
- While mixing the watermelon, add 5-6 fresh mint leaves for a minty-flavored cocktail.
- Choose either red or yellow watermelon.
- Watermelon flavor is sweet and pulpy, with a slight aftertaste of fresh lime.

Serving Suggestions: This juice is a refreshing drink to serve in the afternoon during the hot summer months. It quickly refills bodily water without increasing calorie intake.

*Recipe 8*

## Pears Juice

In Hindi, pears are called as Nashpati. A good number of natives usually eat fruits directly, although I occasionally create fruit juices during my stay there. In just a few minutes, you can produce this simple and delightful pear juice recipe. I'll show you how to produce sweet and healthful pear juice that you can drink on a hot day.

Pear juice has a pleasant taste with a tinge of apple flavor. Although adding ice cubes is optional, cooled juice tastes better. If you don't want to use ice cubes, use cooled water instead.

I recommend incorporating ginger and mint leaves into the juice. Their inclusion, however, is optional.

According to Wikipedia, pears contain 84% water, 15% carbohydrates, and are a rich source of dietary fiber. Include pears in your diet because they are high in nutrients and antioxidants.

*Preparations*:

Rinse and peel 3 to 4 medium to large sized pears.

- Peel and cut the pears.

- Place the pears in a blender jar or juicer.

- Stir in 1/2 tbsp lemon juice. Adding lemon juice avoids juice discoloration and adds a wonderful tang to the drink. If you want to make it more nutritious, add mint leaves or sliced ginger at this stage.

- If you prefer a sweeter flavor, add more sugar or honey, but keep in mind that pear is a sweet fruit. As a result, adjust the sugar proportionately. Pour in the ice cubes.

- If you don't want your juice chilly, use 1/4 cup room temperature water for the ice. You can also substitute cooled water for the ice.

- Puree till smooth.

- Strain the juice through a mesh sieve. You do not need to filter the pear juice if you used a juicer.

- Serve the pear juice in tall glasses right away.

## Recipe 9

### Lemonade Juice Recipe

Make the Best Lemonade Ever when life gives you lemons! This recipe is as fantastic as it gets: sweet, tangy, simple to make, and oh-so-refreshing. Make your best-rated lemonade recipe to brighten your day using these simple steps.

## Ingredients

- 1/2 cups of water
- 1 teaspoon of sugar substitute, such as Stevia
- 1/2 teaspoon lemon or lime peel, finely shredded
- 1/4 cup freshly squeezed lemon or lime juice
- Cubes of ice

## Preparation

- Heat water and sugar or sugar substitute in a medium saucepan over medium heat until sugar is dissolved. Remove from heat and set aside for 20 minutes to cool. (If you're in a hurry, skip the heat. Rather, dissolve the sugar or its substitute in room temperature water before proceeding to step #2.)

- Add citrus peel and juice to sugar or sugar substitute mixture. Cover and refrigerate in a jar or pitcher.. Keeps for up to 3 days.

- In ice-filled glasses, blend 3 ounces base and 3 ounces water for each glass of lemonade or limeade. To enjoy, stir and sip leisurely. Freeze leftover base in ice cube trays and use instead of ice in beverages.

**Helpful Hints**

- 6 tablespoons is 3 ounces of liquid.
- Stevia-sweetened base includes 20 calories and 5 grams of carbs. Count as half of your carbohydrate option.

## *Recipe 10*

**Cherry Juice Recipes**

Cherry juice has a number of health benefits. The most famous of its therapeutic effects are pain relief for rheumatoid arthritis, gout, diabetes, and heart diseases making it a great delight for patients who experience these illness. Aside from red cherries, this recipe also includes plums and watermelon to make the juice more flavorful and appealing.

## Ingredients:

- 15 ripe and fresh red cherries
- 1/2 cup watermelon, diced
- 3 Plums
- 4 cubes of ice

## Preparation:

- Wash the cherries and plums. Remove the cherries' seeds.

- Blanch plums (boil for 2 minutes in hot water, then quickly submerge in cold water for 1 minute) and peel them. Its skin is often rather sour, so it is advised to remove it. If you want a tart flavor, you can use it with the skin on.

- Cut the plums in half and take off the stones.

- In a blender, purée the cherries, watermelon, and plums until smooth.

- Strain the puree through a sieve, collecting the liquid in a basin and removing the watermelon seeds.

- Fill serving glasses with ice cubes and fill with the fruitful and natural juice of red cherry.

**Suggestions and Variations**:

• You may also prepare it with a juicer instead of a blender.

• If the watermelon isn't sweet enough, add 1 teaspoon sugar.

• Use black cherry to generate juice with a stronger flavor.

*Recipe 11*

**Carrot Juice Recipe**

This nutritious drink is refreshing, easy to make, and delicious. The following steps will make your preparation of this fantastic juice quick and easy.

*Ingredients*

• Carrots (500 g)

• 3 tbsp Honey, or to taste

• 3 cups of water

• Ice cubes for serving

• If creating Carrot Orange Juice, add 2 large oranges.

• 1 cucumber (350g) Only use if preparing cucumber carrot juice.

• 2 large apples (optional) if preparing apple carrot juice

• 1 cup of milk Only use for Carrot Juice with Milk.

• 1 inch ginger root for carrot-ginger juice

*Preparation*:

- Remove the outer skin of the carrots or thoroughly wash them to remove any dirt.

- Place carrots in a blender or food processor, followed by water and honey or sugar.

- Blend until smooth, then strain into a basin using a cheesecloth.

- Pour the juice into a pitcher and chill in the refrigerator.

- Serve and Enjoy.

*Recipe 12*

**Celery juice Recipe**

Celery juice is high in vitamins A, C, K, folate, and a variety of other nutrients. Celery juice has also been shown to lower inflammation and is an excellent anti-inflammatory food.

Celery juice has been quite the craze over the last year or two. People have been drinking it as a detox drink because it offers numerous health benefits.

I've been enjoying this fresh celery juice because it's simple to make and tastes delicious. It's seriously excellent and super refreshing.

This celery juice has been a hydrating snack replacement for me, as well as a hunger suppressant. So, if you've been wondering how to create celery juice, let's get started on this nutritious recipe. You will adore this recipe!

Another thing I like about this simple celery juice recipe is that it only requires two ingredients. I know you have one of them, and you may even have the other!

## Ingredients

• Four celery sticks

• 500 mL water

Some celery juice recipes contain sugar, which I believe is absolutely unnecessary and negates the purpose of drinking it. So there's no sugar in this!

## Preparation

• Scrub the celery stalks to eliminate any dirt. Remove the celery stalks' leaves and trim the white ends. Cut the celery into small pieces and combine it with the water in a blender.

• Add water into a blender filled with chopped celery.

- Blend the chopped celery with water until entirely smooth, with no pieces of celery remaining.

- Strain the juices from the pureed celery into a pitcher or glass using a cheesecloth or clean nut milk bag. Serve cool, and drink the celery juice right away.

**Helpful Tips:**

• If you wish to add more flavor, squeeze in some fresh lemon juice.

• To make the recipe even healthier, use organic celery.

• Double or treble the recipe for a week's worth of celery juice.

• If there are still chunks of celery in the blender, add extra water.

• For a more refreshing flavor, serve the celery juice over ice.

*Recipe 13*

**Spinach Juice**

When compared to plain and pure spinach juice, fresh spinach juice blended with apple is significantly more delightful and drinkable. It is well-known for its cleansing properties, as it purifies the blood and eliminates accumulated toxins from the cells, and it also aids in the regeneration and rebuilding of the body. To produce detoxifying juice at home, follow this simple and straightforward method.

*Ingredients*:

• 2 cups tightly packed chopped spinach

• 1 cored and chopped apple or pear

• 1 celery stalk

• 1/2 lime or lemon juice (or to taste), optional

• 3/4 cup of water

*Preparations*:

- Clean the spinach, apple, and celery. Cut the apple and celery into big chunks.

- Fill a blender jar with 3/4 cup water. Mix in the apple and celery.

- Stir in the spinach and lemon juice.

- Blend until smooth in a blender.

- Make sure there are no fruit bits.

- Pour the prepared juice combination into a big container via a fine mesh juice strainer (or sieve).

- Using a spatula, press the pulp down to get as much juice as possible. Remove the pulp.

- Transfer the prepared juice to a serving glass and serve.

**Suggestions and Variations:**

- For the greatest results, use fresh, dark green spinach.
- If you don't like the flavor of spinach alone, combine it with other green veggies such as cucumber, beet, tomato, carrot, and so on to make a delightful nutritious drink.

*Recipe 14*

## Kale Juice

Kale juice should taste as amazing as it feels. With its well-balanced sweet, tangy, spicy, and earthy flavors, this recipe strikes a satisfying chord.

## *Ingredients*

- 2 large curly kale leaves, including stems

- 1/2 cup packed cilantro leaves and stems (14 grams)

- 1 English or Persian cucumber.

- A 12-inch chunk of ginger

- 1 lime

- 1 medium green apple

- 2 celery ribs

## *Preparation*

- Place all ingredients in the juicer in the order mentioned.

- Combine all ingredients and strain through a fine-mesh sieve.

- Transfer to a glass and serve.

## Notes

• Green curly kale has a moderate flavor and produces a large amount of juice. You'll need two huge leaves, as well as the stems.

• Cilantro provides numerous health benefits as well as a strong flavor. What it brings to this juice is fantastic. If you don't like it, you can replace it with parsley.

*Recipe 15*

**Green Zucchini Juice**

Green juices are refreshing and appetizing, as well as a healthy supply of fluid for hydration. This juice has several health benefits, including blood sugar regulation, weight management, bad cholesterol elimination, vision improvement, gout prevention, and cancer prevention.

*Ingredients*

• 1 apple

• 2 (courgette)

• 4 leaves kale (Tuscan cabbage)

• 1 inch (1/2 cm) ginger slice

• ½ lemon

*Preparation*:

- Thoroughly wash all produce.

- Peel the lemon if you prefer a less bitter flavor.

- Juice all of the ingredients in a juicer and enjoy!

*Recipe 16*

**Bok Choy Juice Recipe**

For millennia, the East has employed bok choy kale medicinally. It includes over 70 antioxidants and detoxifies the body while also promoting optimal metabolism and cellular health.

Furthermore, we will be utilizing a highly medicinal produce known as beets. Beet tops and leaves can help with diabetes, anemia, heart disease, and thyroid issues. The apple will sweeten the beverage.

## *Ingredients*:

- 1 small bok choy

- Beets and their greens

- 1 Apple

- 1 fennel bulb

## *Preparation*:

1. Wash the bok choy, beets, and their greens, as well as the apple.

2. Juice the items in a juicer.

3. Serve right away. Enjoy!

*Recipe 17*

**Parsley Juice Recipe**

This Parsley Juice recipe is a nutritious green juice that is high in hydrating nourishment. The invigorating and cleansing benefits of parsley are well known. This green juice can be had in the morning or at any time of day.

*Ingredients*:

• 1 bunch washed and dried flat leaf parsley

• 1 washed and sliced apple (red or green)

• 1 English cucumber, sliced into long slices large enough to fit through your juicer

• 1 lemon, skinned and sliced

*Preparation*

• Prepare vegetables by washing and chopping them so that they will fit into the tube of a masticating juicer.

- Feed the veggies through the tube, alternating between firm and soft textures to aid in the juicing process.

- Serve immediately.

Notes:

• I normally wash the full bunch of parsley under running water before cutting off the bottom third of the stalks to prepare it for juicing. You can juice the parsley leaves and stem.

• For maximum nutrition, fresh juices should be drunk within 24 hours. Any leftovers should be refrigerated in a firmly sealed container.

• BLENDER INSTRUCTIONS: Place the ingredients in the base of a high-speed blender and blend until smooth. To properly combine the ingredients, you may need to add 1/4 to 1/2 cup of water. Process for 30-45 seconds on high. Pour the mixture through a nut milk bag, reserving only the juice. Remove the pulp or keep it for another purpose.

• Pregnant women and individuals taking blood thinners should avoid using this recipe.

## Recipe 18

### Lettuce Juice Recipe

Lettuce juice is a simple approach to hydrate and consume nutrients. You don't even need a juicer to make this simple and nutritious drink.

### Ingredients:

• 4 cups romaine lettuce, chopped

• 1/2 cup green apple, diced

- 1/2 cup cucumber, diced

- 1/2 lemon, skin included

4 cups of purified water

## *Preparation*

- In a blender, combine and blend all of the ingredients.

- Liquify for one minute, or until all of the ingredients are broken down.

- Cover a bigger bowl with a nut milk bag, several layers of cheesecloth, or a thin kitchen towel.

- Empty the contents of the blender into the bowl, straining the pulp with a nut milk bag, cheesecloth, or towel.

- Refrigerate the juice and consume it within two days.

**Notes**

• If using a juicer, simply process everything except the water in the juicer.

*Recipe 19*

**Beet juice Recipe**

Beetroot, a beautiful veggie, promotes cardiovascular health. Beetroot juice has been clinically proved to help lower excessive blood pressure and thereby prevent cardiovascular diseases. Apart from this most noticeable benefit, it has a plethora of other advantages, placing it among the healthiest juice recipes. It's a basic combination of red beet, apple, and celery.

## Ingredients:

- 1 little red beet

- 1 medium (or 2 small) apple

- 2 stalks celery

- 1 or 2 carrots

- Half a lemon or lime

- 1/2 inch tiny piece peeled ginger

## Preparation:

- Wash and pat dry all veggies and fruits under running water.

- Peel the beets and cut it into long pieces. Separate the core from the apple and cut it into long pieces. Peel and chop the carrot into long pieces. Cut the celery into long strips.

- Place a glass or container under the juicer's nozzle and turn it on.

- Juice all ingredients except the lemon (beetroot, apple, carrot, celery, ginger) in a juicer.

- Squeeze half a lemon into the prepared juice and thoroughly mix. Pour into a cold glass and serve. Drink it right away.

## Suggestions and Variations:

• Select a small, firm beetroot. We also used sweet apple, but you can use any variety of apple you want.

• Pure beetroot juice is quite strong; always blend it with another fruit or vegetable juice to reduce the possibility of negative effects.

• If you're using organic vegetables and fruits, do not peel them.

## Recipe 20

**Asparagus Juice Recipe**

Asparagus juice, which is high in critical minerals and antioxidants, provides several health benefits while also tempting your taste senses. These asparagus juice recipes are a must-try if you're eager to test new juicing choices or simply want to integrate more greens into your diet. Prepare to embark on a delectable and healthful adventure with these delectable concoctions!

## Ingredients:

• 1 asparagus bunch

• Two cucumbers

• Two green apples

• 1 lemon

*Preparation*:

- Prepare the asparagus, cucumbers, and apples by washing and trimming them.

- To make blending easier, cut the asparagus spears into smaller pieces.

- Peel and seed the apples before cutting them into wedges.

- Extract the juice from the asparagus, cucumbers, apples, and lemon.

- Stir thoroughly and serve with ice for a cool drink.

*Recipe 21*

## Broccoli Juice Recipe

Broccolis are delicious in a variety of ways, including cheesy casseroles, stir-fries with meat, and freshly steamed with a dipping sauce on the side, to mention a few. With the correct accompaniments, this green vegetable can also be used to make a delicious drink.

The freshly extracted broccoli-spinach elixir is combined with pear juice, lemon juice, mint, and ice in my recipe. The tart-sweet beverage leans toward sweetness and has a refreshing, soothing scent.

Broccoli is high in vitamin C and K, and it also includes vitamin A, vitamin B9, potassium, and phosphorus, among other nutrients. All of these are low in calories, making it a perfect food to eat to feel full and avoid overeating later.

## Ingredients

- 6 oz soaked and cleaned broccoli

- 1 oz soaked and cleaned spinach

- 1 pound pear

- 1 teaspoon lemon juice

- 8 mint leaves

- 1 cup of water

- 2 cups of ice

## Preparation:

- Juice the broccoli, spinach, pear, and mint in a juicer.

- Combine the juice, water, and lemon juice in a mixing bowl.

- Serve with ice.

If you have followed our essential 21-recipe diabetic renal juicing guide to this point, it means you truly care about your diabetic renal health. These juices are specially selected for patients who wish to regulate their blood sugar as well as avoid dialysis as a result of kidney function retardation.

Most patients, after diagnosis, find it challenging to select their meal because of the fear of not knowing what food might likely spike their blood sugar level. I have taken all these into consideration, and in the next chapter (bonus page) of your book, we will be giving out a simple 21-day meal plan that patients can follow.

I hope you are enjoying your read so far. As a token of appreciation, we humbly ask that you drop a review about our book on the website. These reviews can also help us find our next book to meet your personal needs.

# Bonus 1

## 21-Day Diabetic Kidney Disease Meal Plan

Welcome to the 21-day meal plan for diabetic renal patients. With careful consideration of nutritional balance and variety, we present to you this easy 21-day meal plan that will help you regulate your sugar level and retard the progression of kidney disease.

Below is a specially crafted meal plan that incorporates the essential juices that were discussed in the previous chapters of this book. These juices and dishes in this meal plan are proven to offer a balanced diet for each day. Please note that this is a general meal plan, and individual dietary needs may vary. Patients with critical health conditions should consult with a healthcare professional or registered dietitian for personalized guidance.

*WEEK 1*

**Day 1:**

- Breakfast: Cucumber Juice

- Snack: Carrot Sticks with Hummus

- Lunch: Spinach Salad with Grilled Chicken

- Snack: Blueberry Juice

- Dinner: Baked Salmon with Steamed Broccoli

**Day 2:**

- Breakfast: Pineapple Juice

- Snack: Greek Yogurt with Berries

- Lunch: Turkey and Avocado Wrap

- Snack: Celery Juice

- Dinner: Grilled Shrimp with Asparagus

**Day 3:**

- Breakfast: Celery Juice

- Snack: Almonds

- Lunch: Lentil Soup with a Side Salad

- Snack: Cherry Juice

- Dinner: Baked Chicken with Roasted Zucchini

**Day 4:**

- Breakfast: Cranberries Juice

- Snack: Sliced Cucumbers with Cottage Cheese

- Lunch: Quinoa Salad with Chickpeas and Veggies

- Snack: Grape Juice

- Dinner: Baked Cod with Steamed Spinach

**Day 5:**

- Breakfast: Blueberry Juice

- Snack: Celery Sticks with Peanut Butter

- Lunch: Tuna Salad on Whole Grain Bread

- Snack: Lemonade Juice

- Dinner: Grilled Turkey Burger with Lettuce and Tomato

**Day 6:**

- Breakfast: Watermelon Juice

- Snack: Mixed Nuts

- Lunch: Roasted Chicken Breast with Green Beans

- Snack: Pears Juice

- Dinner: Baked Tilapia with Bok Choy

**Day 7:**

- Breakfast: Cherry Juice

- Snack: Sliced Carrots with Hummus

- Lunch: Quinoa and Black Bean Bowl

- Snack: Kale Juice

- Dinner: Stir-Fried Tofu with Broccoli

*WEEK 2*

**Day 8:**

- Breakfast: Pineapple Juice
- Snack: Sliced Cucumbers with Cottage Cheese
- Lunch: Grilled Chicken Salad with Mixed Greens
- Snack: Cranberries Juice

- Dinner: Baked Cod with Steamed Broccoli

**Day 9:**

- Breakfast: Celery Juice
- Snack: Almonds
- Lunch: Turkey and Avocado Wrap
- Snack: Blueberry Juice
- Dinner: Baked Salmon with Roasted Brussels Sprouts

**Day 10:**

- Breakfast: Cucumber Juice
- Snack: Carrot Sticks with Hummus
- Lunch: Quinoa and Black Bean Bowl
- Snack: Grape Juice
- Dinner: Grilled Shrimp with Asparagus

**Day 11:**

- Breakfast: Cherry Juice
- Snack: Mixed Berries and Greek Yogurt
- Lunch: Lentil Soup with a Side Salad
- Snack: Lemonade Juice
- Dinner: Baked Chicken with Sautéed Spinach

**Day 12:**

- Breakfast: Blueberry Juice

- Snack: Sliced Carrots with Peanut Butter

- Lunch: Spinach Salad with Grilled Tofu

- Snack: Parsley Juice

- Dinner: Baked Tilapia with Steamed Green Beans

**Day 13:**

- Breakfast: Watermelon Juice

- Snack: Mixed Nuts

- Lunch: Tuna Salad on Whole Grain Bread

- Snack: Green Zucchini Juice

- Dinner: Stir-Fried Tempeh with Bok Choy

**Day 14:**

- Breakfast: Beet Juice

- Snack: Sliced Bell Peppers with Guacamole

- Lunch: Chickpea and Vegetable Stir-Fry

- Snack: Asparagus Juice

- Dinner: Grilled Turkey Burger with Mixed Greens

# WEEK 3

**Day 15:**

- Breakfast: Beet Juice
- Snack: Sliced Cucumbers with Cottage Cheese
- Lunch: Grilled Vegetable and Quinoa Salad
- Snack: Green Zucchini Juice
- Dinner: Baked Salmon with Lemon and Asparagus

**Day 16:**

- Breakfast: Pears Juice
- Snack: Almonds
- Lunch: Turkey and Avocado Wrap
- Snack: Cranberries Juice
- Dinner: Baked Cod with Steamed Broccoli

**Day 17:**

- Breakfast: Cherry Juice
- Snack: Mixed Berries and Greek Yogurt
- Lunch: Lentil Soup with a Side Salad
- Snack: Celery Juice
- Dinner: Grilled Chicken with Roasted Brussels Sprouts

**Day 18:**

- Breakfast: Blueberry Juice
- Snack: Sliced Carrots with Hummus
- Lunch: Quinoa and Black Bean Bowl
- Snack: Parsley Juice
- Dinner: Baked Tilapia with Sautéed Spinach

**Day 19:**

- Breakfast: Cucumber Juice
- Snack: Walnuts
- Lunch: Spinach Salad with Grilled Shrimp
- Snack: Grape Juice
- Dinner: Baked Chicken with Green Beans

**Day 20:**

- Breakfast: Asparagus Juice
- Snack: Sliced Bell Peppers with Guacamole
- Lunch: Tuna Salad on Whole Grain Bread
- Snack: Lemonade Juice
- Dinner: Grilled Turkey Burger with Steamed Broccoli

**Day 21:**

- Breakfast: Broccoli Juice

- Snack: Cherry Tomatoes with Mozzarella Cheese
- Lunch: Chickpea and Vegetable Stir-Fry
- Snack: Celery Juice
- Dinner: Baked Salmon with Roasted Asparagus

I hope you enjoyed using this comprehensive 21-day meal plan, as it incorporates a variety of juice recipes and kidney-friendly meals to help manage diabetes while supporting renal health. Always remember to adapt portion sizes and food choices based on your specific dietary needs and always try to plan your meals with journals. In the bonus 2 of our book, we will be providing a food journal to help you achieve proper journaling and food planning with ease.

Never hesitate to consult with a healthcare provider or registered dietitian for personalized guidance and adjustments if your health condition is at a critical stage. Note that staying consistent with a balanced diet and monitoring blood sugar levels will be crucial for managing diabetes effectively.

# Conclusion

In conclusion, ***"Diabetic Renal Juicing for Seniors"*** is a comprehensive guide that aims to educate individuals with diabetic renal disease on the benefits of juicing fruits and vegetables for their health. The book provides information on the causes and symptoms of diabetic renal disease, as well as tips for maintaining kidney health. It also emphasizes the importance of preventing type 2 diabetes to avoid kidney disease. The book provides readers with the knowledge and tools to make informed decisions about their health and offers hope for managing diabetes and renal disease through the power of natural juices.

Juicing can be a beneficial addition to the diet for individuals with diabetic kidney disease, as it provides increased concentrations of vitamins, minerals, and phytonutrients. However, it is important to carefully select the right juicer and consider the potential loss of fiber and increased sugar consumption. It is also crucial to be mindful of potassium intake and avoid juicing potassium-rich fruits and vegetables. Low-potassium juices, such as apple, cranberry, and grape juices, can be a good option for individuals with kidney disease.

The bonus chapters of this book provides a 21-day meal plan and a food journal for diabetic renal patients. The meal plan incorporates essential juices discussed in previous chapters and aims to regulate blood sugar levels and slow down the progression of kidney disease as well as a food journal to ensure meals are properly planned and followed with ease.

# Bonus 2

## Food Journal

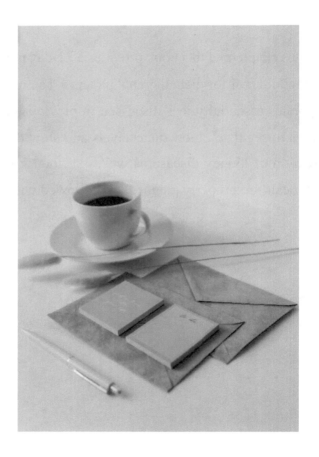

# FOOD JOURNAL

| Breakfast | Servings | Calories |
|---|---|---|
| | | |
| | | |
| | Subtotal | |

| Snack | | |
|---|---|---|
| | | |
| | Subtotal | |

| Lunch | | |
|---|---|---|
| | | |
| | | |
| | Subtotal | |

| Snack | | |
|---|---|---|
| | | |
| | Subtotal | |

| Dinner | | |
|---|---|---|
| | | |
| | | |
| | Subtotal | |

| Snack | | |
|---|---|---|
| | | |
| | Subtotal | |

**Total Calories From Food**

## FITNESS ACTIVITY JOURNAL

| | Duration | Calories |
|---|---|---|
| | | |
| | | |
| | | |

**Total Calories From Fitness**

## NOTES

# FOOD JOURNAL

| Breakfast | Servings | Calories |
|---|---|---|
| | | |
| | | |
| | | |
| | Subtotal | |

| Snack | | |
|---|---|---|
| | | |
| | Subtotal | |

| Lunch | | |
|---|---|---|
| | | |
| | | |
| | | |
| | Subtotal | |

| Snack | | |
|---|---|---|
| | | |
| | Subtotal | |

| Dinner | | |
|---|---|---|
| | | |
| | | |
| | | |
| | Subtotal | |

| Snack | | |
|---|---|---|
| | | |
| | Subtotal | |

**Total Calories From Food**

## FITNESS ACTIVITY JOURNAL

| | Duration | Calories |
|---|---|---|
| | | |
| | | |
| | | |
| | | |

**Total Calories From Fitness**

## NOTES

# FOOD JOURNAL

| Breakfast | Servings | Calories |
|---|---|---|
|  |  |  |
|  |  |  |
|  |  |  |
|  | Subtotal |  |

| Snack | | |
|---|---|---|
|  |  |  |
|  | Subtotal |  |

| Lunch | | |
|---|---|---|
|  |  |  |
|  |  |  |
|  |  |  |
|  | Subtotal |  |

| Snack | | |
|---|---|---|
|  |  |  |
|  | Subtotal |  |

| Dinner | | |
|---|---|---|
|  |  |  |
|  |  |  |
|  |  |  |
|  | Subtotal |  |

| Snack | | |
|---|---|---|
|  |  |  |
|  | Subtotal |  |

**Total Calories From Food**

## FITNESS ACTIVITY JOURNAL

| | Duration | Calories |
|---|---|---|
|  |  |  |
|  |  |  |
|  |  |  |

**Total Calories From Fitness**

## NOTES

# FOOD JOURNAL

| Breakfast | Servings | Calories |
|---|---|---|
| | | |
| | | |
| | | |
| | Subtotal | |

| Snack | | |
|---|---|---|
| | | |
| | Subtotal | |

| Lunch | | |
|---|---|---|
| | | |
| | | |
| | | |
| | Subtotal | |

| Snack | | |
|---|---|---|
| | | |
| | Subtotal | |

| Dinner | | |
|---|---|---|
| | | |
| | | |
| | | |
| | Subtotal | |

| Snack | | |
|---|---|---|
| | | |
| | Subtotal | |

| | Total Calories From Food | |
|---|---|---|

## FITNESS ACTIVITY JOURNAL

| | Duration | Calories |
|---|---|---|
| | | |
| | | |
| | | |
| | | |
| | Total Calories From Fitness | |

## NOTES

# FOOD JOURNAL

| Breakfast | Servings | Calories |
|---|---|---|
|  |  |  |
|  |  |  |
|  |  |  |
|  | Subtotal |  |

| Snack |  |  |
|---|---|---|
|  |  |  |
|  | Subtotal |  |

| Lunch |  |  |
|---|---|---|
|  |  |  |
|  |  |  |
|  | Subtotal |  |

| Snack |  |  |
|---|---|---|
|  |  |  |
|  | Subtotal |  |

| Dinner |  |  |
|---|---|---|
|  |  |  |
|  |  |  |
|  | Subtotal |  |

| Snack |  |  |
|---|---|---|
|  |  |  |
|  | Subtotal |  |

**Total Calories From Food** [          ]

## FITNESS ACTIVITY JOURNAL

|  | Duration | Calories |
|---|---|---|
|  |  |  |
|  |  |  |
|  |  |  |

**Total Calories From Fitness** [          ]

## NOTES

# FOOD JOURNAL

| Breakfast | Servings | Calories |
|---|---|---|
| | | |
| | | |
| | | |
| | Subtotal | |

| Snack | | |
|---|---|---|
| | | |
| | Subtotal | |

| Lunch | | |
|---|---|---|
| | | |
| | | |
| | | |
| | Subtotal | |

| Snack | | |
|---|---|---|
| | | |
| | Subtotal | |

| Dinner | | |
|---|---|---|
| | | |
| | | |
| | | |
| | Subtotal | |

| Snack | | |
|---|---|---|
| | | |
| | Subtotal | |

**Total Calories From Food** [ ]

## FITNESS ACTIVITY JOURNAL

| | Duration | Calories |
|---|---|---|
| | | |
| | | |
| | | |
| | | |

**Total Calories From Fitness** [ ]

## NOTES

# FOOD JOURNAL

| Breakfast | Servings | Calories |
|---|---|---|
| | | |
| | | |
| | Subtotal | |
| **Snack** | | |
| | Subtotal | |
| **Lunch** | | |
| | | |
| | Subtotal | |
| **Snack** | | |
| | Subtotal | |
| **Dinner** | | |
| | | |
| | Subtotal | |
| **Snack** | | |
| | Subtotal | |

Total Calories From Food [＿＿＿＿＿＿]

## FITNESS ACTIVITY JOURNAL

| | Duration | Calories |
|---|---|---|
| | | |
| | | |
| | | |

Total Calories From Fitness [＿＿＿＿＿＿]

## NOTES

# FOOD JOURNAL

| Breakfast | Servings | Calories |
|---|---|---|
| | | |
| | | |
| | | |
| | Subtotal | |

| Snack | | |
|---|---|---|
| | | |
| | Subtotal | |

| Lunch | | |
|---|---|---|
| | | |
| | | |
| | | |
| | Subtotal | |

| Snack | | |
|---|---|---|
| | | |
| | Subtotal | |

| Dinner | | |
|---|---|---|
| | | |
| | | |
| | | |
| | Subtotal | |

| Snack | | |
|---|---|---|
| | | |
| | Subtotal | |

**Total Calories From Food** [          ]

## FITNESS ACTIVITY JOURNAL

| | Duration | Calories |
|---|---|---|
| | | |
| | | |
| | | |

**Total Calories From Fitness** [          ]

## NOTES

# FOOD JOURNAL

| Breakfast | Servings | Calories |
|---|---|---|
|  |  |  |
|  |  |  |
|  |  |  |
|  | Subtotal |  |

| Snack | | |
|---|---|---|
|  |  |  |
|  | Subtotal |  |

| Lunch | | |
|---|---|---|
|  |  |  |
|  |  |  |
|  |  |  |
|  | Subtotal |  |

| Snack | | |
|---|---|---|
|  |  |  |
|  | Subtotal |  |

| Dinner | | |
|---|---|---|
|  |  |  |
|  |  |  |
|  |  |  |
|  | Subtotal |  |

| Snack | | |
|---|---|---|
|  |  |  |
|  | Subtotal |  |

**Total Calories From Food**

## FITNESS ACTIVITY JOURNAL

| | Duration | Calories |
|---|---|---|
|  |  |  |
|  |  |  |
|  |  |  |
|  |  |  |

**Total Calories From Fitness**

## NOTES

# FOOD JOURNAL

| Breakfast | | Servings | Calories |
|---|---|---|---|
| | | | |
| | | | |
| | | | |
| | | Subtotal | |

| Snack | | | |
|---|---|---|---|
| | | | |
| | | Subtotal | |

| Lunch | | | |
|---|---|---|---|
| | | | |
| | | | |
| | | | |
| | | Subtotal | |

| Snack | | | |
|---|---|---|---|
| | | | |
| | | Subtotal | |

| Dinner | | | |
|---|---|---|---|
| | | | |
| | | | |
| | | | |
| | | Subtotal | |

| Snack | | | |
|---|---|---|---|
| | | | |
| | | Subtotal | |

Total Calories From Food [           ]

## FITNESS ACTIVITY JOURNAL

| | Duration | Calories |
|---|---|---|
| | | |
| | | |
| | | |
| | | |

Total Calories From Fitness [           ]

## NOTES

# FOOD JOURNAL

| Breakfast | Servings | Calories |
|---|---|---|
|  |  |  |
|  |  |  |
|  | Subtotal |  |

| Snack | | |
|---|---|---|
|  |  |  |
|  | Subtotal |  |

| Lunch | | |
|---|---|---|
|  |  |  |
|  |  |  |
|  | Subtotal |  |

| Snack | | |
|---|---|---|
|  |  |  |
|  | Subtotal |  |

| Dinner | | |
|---|---|---|
|  |  |  |
|  |  |  |
|  | Subtotal |  |

| Snack | | |
|---|---|---|
|  |  |  |
|  | Subtotal |  |

**Total Calories From Food**

## FITNESS ACTIVITY JOURNAL

| | Duration | Calories |
|---|---|---|
|  |  |  |
|  |  |  |
|  |  |  |

**Total Calories From Fitness**

## NOTES

# FOOD JOURNAL

| Breakfast | Servings | Calories | |
|---|---|---|---|
| | | | |
| | | | |
| | | Subtotal | |

| Snack | | | |
|---|---|---|---|
| | | | |
| | | Subtotal | |

| Lunch | | | |
|---|---|---|---|
| | | | |
| | | | |
| | | | |
| | | Subtotal | |

| Snack | | | |
|---|---|---|---|
| | | | |
| | | Subtotal | |

| Dinner | | | |
|---|---|---|---|
| | | | |
| | | | |
| | | | |
| | | Subtotal | |

| Snack | | | |
|---|---|---|---|
| | | | |
| | | Subtotal | |

Total Calories From Food [            ]

**FITNESS ACTIVITY JOURNAL**

| | Duration | Calories |
|---|---|---|
| | | |
| | | |
| | | |
| | | |

Total Calories From Fitness [            ]

**NOTES**

# FOOD JOURNAL

| Breakfast | Servings | Calories | |
|---|---|---|---|
| | | | |
| | | | |
| | | Subtotal | |
| **Snack** | | | |
| | | Subtotal | |
| **Lunch** | | | |
| | | | |
| | | | |
| | | Subtotal | |
| **Snack** | | | |
| | | Subtotal | |
| **Dinner** | | | |
| | | | |
| | | | |
| | | Subtotal | |
| **Snack** | | | |
| | | Subtotal | |

**Total Calories From Food**

## FITNESS ACTIVITY JOURNAL

| | Duration | Calories |
|---|---|---|
| | | |
| | | |
| | | |

**Total Calories From Fitness**

## NOTES

# FOOD JOURNAL

| Breakfast | Servings | Calories | |
|---|---|---|---|
| | | | |
| | | | |
| | | Subtotal | |

| Snack | | | |
|---|---|---|---|
| | | | |
| | | Subtotal | |

| Lunch | | | |
|---|---|---|---|
| | | | |
| | | | |
| | | Subtotal | |

| Snack | | | |
|---|---|---|---|
| | | | |
| | | Subtotal | |

| Dinner | | | |
|---|---|---|---|
| | | | |
| | | | |
| | | Subtotal | |

| Snack | | | |
|---|---|---|---|
| | | | |
| | | Subtotal | |

Total Calories From Food

## FITNESS ACTIVITY JOURNAL

| | Duration | Calories |
|---|---|---|
| | | |
| | | |
| | | |

Total Calories From Fitness

## NOTES

# FOOD JOURNAL

| Breakfast | Servings | Calories |
|---|---|---|
| | | |
| | | |
| | Subtotal | |

| Snack | | |
|---|---|---|
| | Subtotal | |

| Lunch | | |
|---|---|---|
| | | |
| | | |
| | Subtotal | |

| Snack | | |
|---|---|---|
| | Subtotal | |

| Dinner | | |
|---|---|---|
| | | |
| | | |
| | Subtotal | |

| Snack | | |
|---|---|---|
| | Subtotal | |

Total Calories From Food

FITNESS ACTIVITY JOURNAL

| | Duration | Calories |
|---|---|---|
| | | |
| | | |
| | | |

Total Calories From Fitness

NOTES

# FOOD JOURNAL

| Breakfast | Servings | Calories | |
|---|---|---|---|
| | | | |
| | | | |
| | | Subtotal | |

| Snack | | | |
|---|---|---|---|
| | | | |
| | | Subtotal | |

| Lunch | | | |
|---|---|---|---|
| | | | |
| | | | |
| | | | |
| | | Subtotal | |

| Snack | | | |
|---|---|---|---|
| | | | |
| | | Subtotal | |

| Dinner | | | |
|---|---|---|---|
| | | | |
| | | | |
| | | | |
| | | Subtotal | |

| Snack | | | |
|---|---|---|---|
| | | | |
| | | Subtotal | |

Total Calories From Food

**FITNESS ACTIVITY JOURNAL**

| | Duration | Calories |
|---|---|---|
| | | |
| | | |
| | | |
| | | |

Total Calories From Fitness

**NOTES**

# FOOD JOURNAL

| Breakfast | Servings | Calories |
|---|---|---|
|  |  |  |
|  |  |  |
|  | Subtotal |  |

| Snack | | |
|---|---|---|
|  |  |  |
|  | Subtotal |  |

| Lunch | | |
|---|---|---|
|  |  |  |
|  |  |  |
|  |  |  |
|  | Subtotal |  |

| Snack | | |
|---|---|---|
|  |  |  |
|  | Subtotal |  |

| Dinner | | |
|---|---|---|
|  |  |  |
|  |  |  |
|  |  |  |
|  | Subtotal |  |

| Snack | | |
|---|---|---|
|  |  |  |
|  | Subtotal |  |

**Total Calories From Food**

## FITNESS ACTIVITY JOURNAL

| | Duration | Calories |
|---|---|---|
|  |  |  |
|  |  |  |
|  |  |  |

**Total Calories From Fitness**

## NOTES

# FOOD JOURNAL

| Breakfast | Servings | Calories |
|---|---|---|
|  |  |  |
|  |  |  |
|  |  |  |
|  | Subtotal |  |

| Snack | | |
|---|---|---|
|  |  |  |
|  | Subtotal |  |

| Lunch | | |
|---|---|---|
|  |  |  |
|  |  |  |
|  | Subtotal |  |

| Snack | | |
|---|---|---|
|  |  |  |
|  | Subtotal |  |

| Dinner | | |
|---|---|---|
|  |  |  |
|  |  |  |
|  | Subtotal |  |

| Snack | | |
|---|---|---|
|  |  |  |
|  | Subtotal |  |

**Total Calories From Food**

## FITNESS ACTIVITY JOURNAL

| | Duration | Calories |
|---|---|---|
|  |  |  |
|  |  |  |
|  |  |  |
|  |  |  |

**Total Calories From Fitness**

## NOTES

# FOOD JOURNAL

| Breakfast | Servings | Calories |
|---|---|---|
| | | |
| | | |
| | Subtotal | |

| Snack | | |
|---|---|---|
| | Subtotal | |

| Lunch | | |
|---|---|---|
| | | |
| | | |
| | Subtotal | |

| Snack | | |
|---|---|---|
| | Subtotal | |

| Dinner | | |
|---|---|---|
| | | |
| | | |
| | Subtotal | |

| Snack | | |
|---|---|---|
| | Subtotal | |

**Total Calories From Food** [ ]

## FITNESS ACTIVITY JOURNAL

| | Duration | Calories |
|---|---|---|
| | | |
| | | |
| | | |

**Total Calories From Fitness** [ ]

## NOTES

# Picture Links

https://www.pexels.com/photo/blueberries-on-person-s-hand-beside-juice-in-glass-beetroot-and-cucumber-4443483/

https://images.pexels.com/photos/3987343/pexels-photo-3987343.jpeg?auto=compress&cs=tinysrgb&w=600&lazy=load

https://pixabay.com/photos/herbs-smoothies-juice-vegetables-3809512/

https://cdn.pixabay.com/photo/2020/03/22/18/34/dessert-4958151_640.jpg

https://images.pexels.com/photos/4663898/pexels-photo-4663898.jpeg?auto=compress&cs=tinysrgb&w=600&lazy=load

https://images.pexels.com/photos/11009208/pexels-photo-11009208.jpeg?auto=compress&cs=tinysrgb&w=600&lazy=load

Made in United States
Troutdale, OR
01/08/2024

16819621R00070